YOUR KNOWLEDGE HAS VALUE

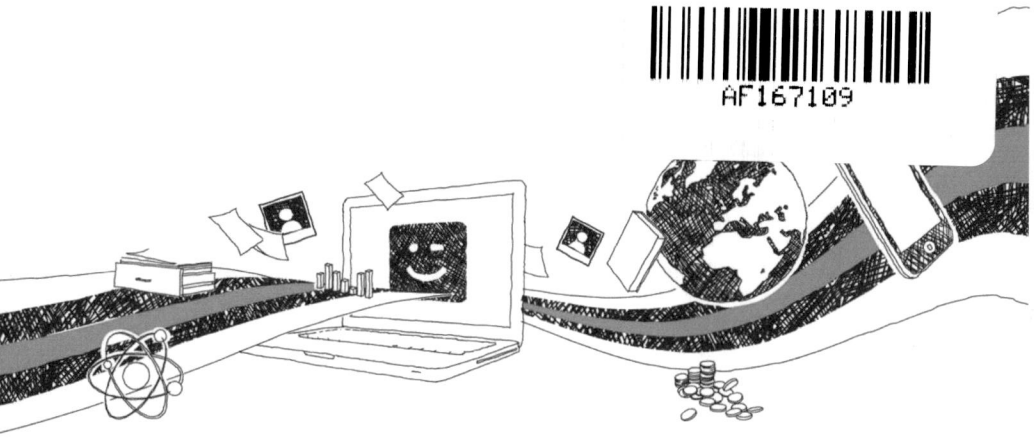
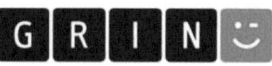

The NotBurger. Meat Substitution by the Use of Methyl Cellulose

Naomi Albiez

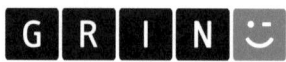

Bibliographic information published by the German National Library:

The German National Library lists this publication in the National Bibliography; detailed bibliographic data are available on the Internet at http://dnb.dnb.de.

ISBN: 9783346794116
This book is also available as an ebook.

© GRIN Publishing GmbH
Nymphenburger Straße 86
80636 München

Print and binding: Books on Demand GmbH, Norderstedt, Germany
Printed on acid-free paper from responsible sources.

The present work has been carefully prepared. Nevertheless, authors and publishers do not incur liability for the correctness of information, notes, links and advice as well as any printing errors.

GRIN web shop: https://www.grin.com/document/1306130

Universidad de Talca - School of Agronomy

Semester Project Report
"NotBurger - Substitution of methyl cellulose".

Author: Naomi Anouk Albiez

02. November 2022

Module: Sensory analysis for product development

Content

1. Introduction

Due to the steady growth of the world's population and increasing wealth in developing countries, the demand for protein is rising (Vázquez-Rowe, 2020). However, it is difficult to meet the demand for protein with animal protein alone. In addition, several customers attach great importance to their well-being and health, so they avoid eating meat for ecological, ethical and social reasons.

On the food industry side, a trend is emerging towards the production of plant-based protein-rich products for human consumption. In the first quarter of 2020, sales of meat substitutes in Germany increased by 37% compared to the first quarter of 2019, from just under 14.7 thousand tons to 20 thousand tons. (Statistisches Bundesamt, 2020)

For consumers to opt for the plant-based alternative, these products must mimic the techno-functional and sensory properties of animal products. In recent years, the offer from different manufacturers has increased and vegan sausages, hamburgers or chicken fillets are already widespread. As soy protein is increasingly rejected by consumers due to concerns about rainforest deforestation and genetically modified seeds, the number of products based on pea or wheat protein is increasing.

Consumers are also increasingly turning their attention to other ingredients, which is why the trend is moving towards "clean labeling". Here, recipes are adapted so that as many, and ideally all, ingredients as possible can be found in the home kitchen. The aim is to counteract the reputation that substitute products are purely chemical and unhealthy foods.

However, substitutes must have the same properties in texture, taste and color as the original ingredients. As this is often based on complex interrelationships, the substitution of methyl cellulose for flaxseed meal in a vegan hamburger will be considered individually in the course of this work. For this purpose, a sensory tasting including the recruitment of panelists and the presentation of samples will be developed.

2. The company „NotCo"

The Santiago, Chile-based start-up "NotCo" specializes in the production of vegan substitute products. Its product range includes plant-based milk and ice cream, as well as vegan burgers. After its founding in 2015, the company expanded first to Brazil and then to all of Latin America, as well as to the United States of America. Since 2021, "NotMeat" has been available in the Chilean branches of BurgerKing and Papa John`s Pizzeria as part of the vegan options. (Wikipedia, 2022)

Editor's note: the figure was removed due to copyright issues.

FIGURE 1: THE LOGO OF "NOTCO" (NOTCO, 2022)

"NotCo" appears on Fast Company's annual list of the world's most innovative companies. (Hassan, 2021) This can be attributed, among other things, to the financial support of investors The Craftory and Jeff Bezos' Bezos Expeditions. However, since 2021 there has been a legal dispute between the Los Rios region's milk producers' union for unfair competition. The union accuses the foodtech company of presenting its product "NotMilk" as a milk substitute and of launching a campaign to position milk as a health food whose production pollutes the environment. For the time being, NotCo defends its right to use the term "milk" for its plant-based drink. (Wikipedia, 2022)

New product development is based on an algorithm patented in 2021. Named "Guiseppe" for marketing reasons, the artificial intelligence contains knowledge of thousands of possible ingredients of plant origin and their combinations. This allows possible recipes to mimic the taste, texture and cooking properties of animal products in a very short time. Machine learning makes it possible to develop ever faster, more efficient and more accurate products. For example, after developing a recipe for a falsely green milk, "Guiseppe" learned that adding dill affects the color of the product and will take this into account in future developments. (NotCo, 2022)

3. The product "NotBurger"

Among vegan meat substitutes, the hamburger remains the most common. Compared to a conventional meat burger, the production of the "NotBurger" requires 89% less energy and 87% less water and generates 89% less CO_2. (NotCo, 2022) These environmental advantages are leading more and more consumers to switch to the vegetable alternative. Therefore, for a better understanding, the following chapter will detail the basics of the recipe and ingredients, as well as the processing. Finally, the requirements for protective packaging will be mentioned.

3.1.Formulation

The hamburger recipe is free of lactose, eggs, soy and genetically modified organisms. Therefore, pea protein extrudates serve as the base. They are created by mixing water with pea protein powder in an extruder. This basic process is discussed in more detail in a later chapter of this report. More ingredients can be found in Figure 2.

INGREDIENTS

Water, Textured pea protein, Coconut oil, Sunflower oil, Natural flavor, Bamboo fiber, Methylcellulose, Pea protein, Yeast extract, Rice protein, Salt, Cocoa powder (processed with alkali), Potato fiber, Psyllium husk, Red beet juice powder (color), Chia protein concentrate, Spinach powder.

FIGURE 2: THE INGREDIENTS OF "NOTBURGER" (NOTCO, 2022)

Coconut oil and sunflower oil contribute to juiciness and fullness in the mouth. Bamboo and potato fibers, as well as methyl cellulose, ensure the cohesion of the dough. To bring the nutritional values closer to those of meat, chia, pea and rice proteins are added for a higher protein content. To achieve a meat-like color, a mixture of cocoa powder, beet powder and spinach powder is added. Finally, a meat-like flavor is achieved thanks to natural flavorings and yeast extract. The different ingredients for the same purpose can be explained by the complexity of the meat, since a specific property can only be achieved by several individual properties of the vegetable ingredients.

3.2. Origen of the raw materials

Since the "NotBurger" is a vegan product, composed only of ingredients of vegetable origin, it should not contain any ingredients of animal origin. All raw materials are of natural origin, the only artificial ingredient is methyl cellulose. In the European market, it bears the designation "E461" and therefore belongs to the additives according to European food legislation. Chemically, methyl cellulose is a cellulose ether, i.e. a compound produced synthetically from cellulose. At room temperature, cellulose is solid. The substance is soluble in cold water. In addition to its use as a food additive, methyl cellulose is found in cosmetic products and paste. The cellulose for the production of the additive is usually sourced from the cotton industry. (Fischer, 2020)

Therefore, the product development task is to replace the only artificial ingredient with an ingredient of natural origin. Since methyl cellulose is used for its binding properties, Linum usitatissimum seed, also known as flaxseed in everyday language, was chosen as a substitute. The flower of the plant can be seen in Figure 3. In order to use the binder properties, ground flaxseed must be used, which after a short time in contact with water turns into a gel. This is to hold the patty dough together.

Editor's note: the figure was removed due to copyright issues.

FIGURE 3: FLOWER OF *LINUM USITATISSIMUM* (GARDENIA , 2023)

The vegetable proteins listed in the ingredient list are created by extracting the proteins from their natural sources using various solvents. This extract is dried and ground into a powder. (Wang, Johnson, & Wang, 2004) More precise information on the natural flavors generally declared cannot be given due to secrecy.

3.3. Production process

Since pea protein extrudates serve as the base and essential contributor to the texture of the veggie burger, the extrusion process is briefly discussed below.

Within a device, proteins are plasticized, mixed, heated, sheared and forced through a die to obtain the desired properties and functionalities of the product. During this process, the biopolymers are subjected to temperatures up to 200 °C and shear rates up to 5000 s^{-1}. (Wittek, Zeiler, Karbstein, & Emin, 2020) Due to heating and shearing during the extrusion process, the macromolecules of food ingredients lose their native structure, resulting in protein denaturation or, in the case of starch, starch gelatinization. The possible extrusion parameters can be classified into three groups, namely process parameters (moisture content, screw configuration, die size, etc.), system parameters (energy input, residence time, etc.) and product characteristics (color, nutritional value, texture, flavor, etc.). (Chen, Wei, Zhang, & Ojokoh, 2010).

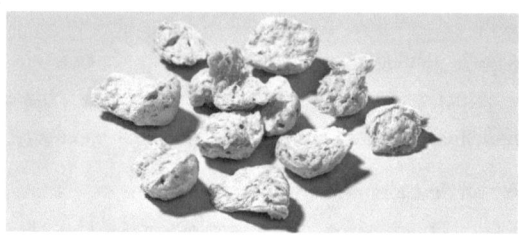

FIGURE 4: EXTRUDED PEA PROTEIN (OWN ILLUSTRATION)

The finished extrudates can be seen in Figure 4. As high temperatures affect the dough in an extruder, colorants and flavorings are only added after the process. This is done by mixing the extrudates with the rest of the ingredients. After shaping and pressing, the patties are frozen at -40 °C to ensure a long shelf life.

Shelf life is defined as the time that elapses from the time it begins to lose its organoleptic properties until it is no longer recommended for consumption. In the case of frozen vegetable products, an expiration date of 6 to 12 months can be expected. An airtight container should be chosen, otherwise the risk of freezer burn increases. This is not dangerous, but the affected foods lose flavor and nutrients. In addition, the affected areas can no longer absorb water during thawing. Therefore, frozen foods lose more flavor and their consistency becomes hard. Frozen products should be stored at - 18 °C. (Vogt & Teichmann, 2021)

In the last step, the patties are individually packaged. There should be as little air space as possible to avoid freezer burn and to save packaging waste. Polyethylene terephthalate (PET) and polyethylene (PE) multilayer packaging systems are suitable for this purpose. PET has good barrier properties against water condensation, while PE has high elasticity and resistance to puncture and frost. This flexible packaging can withstand sub-zero temperatures without losing its quality and durability. The packaging materials guarantee excellent protection against all environmental influences, especially atmospheric gases and moisture. (Uniflex, 2022)

As methyl cellulose is a binder with low nutritional values, the nutritional composition will change only insignificantly. Due to the high fiber content of flaxseed, the energy content may vary marginally upwards. However, as the percentage of methyl cellulose or flaxseed is also low, the table of nutritional values in Figure 5 can be taken from the original product.

Nutrition Facts

4 servings per container

Serving size   1 Patty (113g)

Amount per serving	
Calories	**270**

	% Daily Value*
Total Fat 21g	**27%**
Saturated Fat 13g	**65%**
Trans Fat 0g	
Cholesterol 0mg	**0%**
Sodium 470 mg	**20%**
Total Carbohydrate 8g	**3%**
Dietary Fiber 6g	**21%**
Total Sugars 1g	
Includes 0g Added Sugars	**0%**
Protein 16g	**18%**
Vitamin D 0mcg	0%
Calcium 30mg	2%
Iron 3.6mg	20%
Potassium 350mg	8%
Thiamin 0.12mg	10%
Riboflavin 0.71mg	50%
Niacin 4.1mg	25%
Vitamin B6 0.27mg	15%
Vitamin B12 1.2mcg	50%
Pantothenic Acid 1.2mg	25%
Zinc 4.2mg	40%

The % Daily Value (DV) tells you how much a nutrient in a serving of food contributes to a daily diet. 2,000 calories a day is used for general

FIGURE 5: NUTRITION FACTS PER SERVING (NOTCO, 2022)

4. Modification

The aim of replacing methyl cellulose with flaxseed is to ensure the absence of additives in the product. Although methyl cellulose has the ideal properties as a binder, the trend in the European market, among others, is increasingly towards "clean labeling". This means that certain ingredients are announced on the packaging as not being part of the recipe. (Lebensmittelverband Deutschland, 2022) This also includes the claim "no additives". In the long term, natural flavorings will also be replaced, but the first step is to test whether replacing methyl cellulose with flaxseed makes a significant difference to the product.

The challenge here is that the original product remains unchanged. On the one hand, it concerns the frying properties, which can be tested internally in the "NotCo" test kitchen. The sensory attributes, on the other hand, are to be tested by a consumer panel. The aim is to find out whether there is a significant change in color or texture, or whether the flaxseeds bring their own flavor to the burger.

5. Sensory analysis

By replacing methyl cellulose with flaxseed, there is no change in the product, only the replacement of an artificial ingredient with a natural ingredient. This should not make any noticeable difference in color, texture and taste to the consumer. This now needs to be checked by sensory testing. To detect differences between two samples, the triangle test is suitable. This is a procedure to determine whether there is a sensory perceptible difference or similarity between two samples (A and B). The participant is presented with three coded samples, two the same and one different. In this case, the focus is not on a single attribute, but on the difference of the whole product. A number of 20 - 40 participants, who can be consumers or experts, is recommended. (Moggia, 2022)

5.1.Selection of evaluators and preparations

Since it has to be determined whether the buyer notices the difference, regular consumers of the product have to be recruited for the tasting. This is done through an appeal on social media through the "NotCo" channels. Consumers of the "NotBurger" who live in Santiago will have the opportunity to apply. A product package will be offered as a reward. Through a short application form, suitable participants will be selected to create a consumer panel of 36 participants.

Before arriving, basic rules, such as not using perfumes or strong-smelling soaps, must be explained to the participants. In total, there will be six time slots of 20 minutes each in an afternoon, each with six participants doing the tasting. A larger number of participants per time slot is not recommended, otherwise there will not be enough time to deal with the individual questions. In between, a 10-minute break is foreseen to exchange samples and for the next participants to take their place. The result is a full day's work for the entire tasting. This is because, in addition to the three-hour tasting time, there is also time for sample preparation, set-up and dismantling. Four employees are expected to be responsible for the simultaneous preparation and tasting of the samples. (Navarro, 2022)

The tastings will take place in the company's tasting rooms in Santiago de Chile. They are characterized by separating the preparation area and the tasting booths. The room where the tasting booths are located must be close to the preparation room so that the samples can be brought to the participants quickly and without losing the desired temperature (28 - 30 °C). The lighting is uniform and without shadows, and the room is kept in neutral colors and free of odors and noise. The temperature in the tasting booths is a pleasant 20 - 22 °C and the humidity is 60 - 70%. The layout of the tasting booths can be seen in Figure 6.

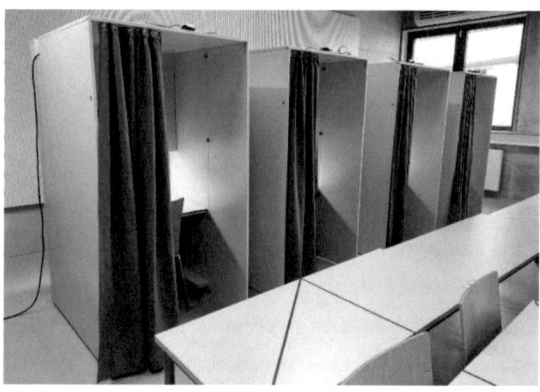

FIGURE 6: EXEMPLARY CONSTRUCION OF TASTING BOOTHS (OWN ILLUSTRATION)

There are six different possibilities to organize the three samples per panelist: AAB, ABA, BAA, BBA, BAB, ABB. To obtain a symmetrical evaluation, a number of panelists is chosen that is a multiple of six. Since each panelist receives three samples, 108 samples have to be prepared. In each case, 54 samples of the original formulation with methylcellulose and 54 samples of the new formulation with linseed. The amount of sample presented should not satiate the subject, so half a hamburger (50 g) divided into three pieces per sample is served. It is also important that the product has the same size and is arranged in the same way each time. (Navarro, 2022)

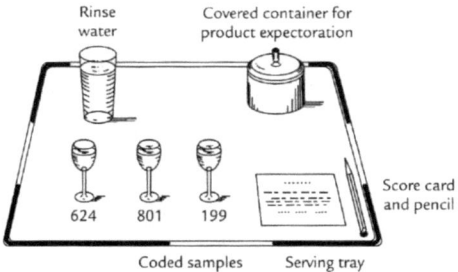

Rinse water
Covered container for product expectoration
Score card and pencil
624   801   199
Coded samples   Serving tray

FIGURE 7: EXEMPLARY PRESENTATION OF SAMPLES IN A TRIANGLE TEST (NAVARRO, 2022)

Figure 7 shows an example of the presentation of the samples. Three coded samples can be seen. However, a total of four three-digit random numbers are needed, since twice A and twice B are tasted among all participants. In addition, a glass of water should be provided to neutralize the taste between tasting the samples. The evaluation sheet and a pen are also provided. Figure 8 shows an exemplary evaluation sheet. (Navarro, 2022) In this case, it is not necessary to provide allergen information, as the product does not contain any allergens.

Triangle Test — Test Code:

Taster No. _____ Name: _____ Date: _____
Type of Sample: _____

Instructions
Taste the samples on the tray from left to right. Two samples are identical; one is different. Select the odd/different sample and indicate by placing an X next to the code of the odd sample.

Samples on tray	Indicate odd sample	Remarks
586	☐	
293	☐	
951	☒	

If you wish to comment on the reasons for your choice or if you wish to comment on the product characteristics, you may do so under Remarks.

FIGURE 8: EXAMPLE OF QUESTIONNAIRE FOR THE EVALUATION (NAVARRO, 2022)

Once the panelists have read and understood the instructions, they can begin to evaluate the samples from left to right. Once the tasting is finished, the questionnaires are placed in an opaque box to preserve the anonymity of the participants.

5.3. Evaluation of results

When evaluating the tests, it is determined how many participants recognized the deviant sample. A table (Figure 9) shows whether this number indicates a significant difference. N in this case means the total number of participants. For the present study, a probability of error of 5 % ($\alpha = 0.05$) is assumed. Therefore, at least 18 participants would have to have correctly recognized the deviant sample.

TABLE T7
Triangle Test for Difference: Critical Number (Minimum) of Correct Answers

Entries are the minimum number of correct responses required for significance at the stated significance level (i.e., column) for the corresponding number of respondents "n" (i.e., row). Reject the assumption of "no difference" if the number of correct responses is greater than or equal to the tabled value.

n	Significance level (%) 10	5	1	0.1	n	Significance level (%) 10	5	1	0.1
3	3	3	—	—	26	13	14	15	17
4	4	4	—	—	27	13	14	16	18
5	4	4	5	—	28	14	15	16	18
					29	14	15	17	19
					30	14	15	17	19
6	5	5	6	—	31	15	16	18	20
7	5	5	6	7	32	15	16	18	20
8	5	6	7	8	33	15	17	18	21
9	6	6	7	8	34	16	17	19	21
10	6	7	8	9	35	16	17	19	22
11	7	7	8	10	36	17	18	20	22
12	7	8	9	10	42	19	20	22	25
13	8	8	9	11	48	21	22	25	27
14	8	9	10	11	54	23	25	27	30
15	8	9	10	12	60	26	27	30	33
16	9	9	11	12	66	28	29	32	35
17	9	10	11	13	72	30	32	34	38
18	10	10	12	13	78	32	34	37	40
19	10	11	12	14	84	35	36	39	43
20	10	11	13	14	90	37	38	42	45
21	11	12	13	15	96	39	41	44	48
22	11	12	14	15					
23	12	12	14	16					
24	12	13	15	16					
25	12	13	15	17					

Note: For values of n not in the table compute $z = (k - (^1/_3)n)/\sqrt{(^2/_9)n}$, where k is the number of correct answers. Compare the computed value of z to the critical value of a standard normal random variable, i.e., the values in the last row of Table T4 ($z_\alpha = t_{\infty,\alpha}$).

FIGURE 9: TRIANGLE TEST: CRITICAL NUMBER OF CORRECT ANSWERS (NAVARRO, 2022)

The null hypothesis H0 is assumed to be "No difference". If more than 18 participants correctly detect a difference, the null hypothesis is rejected and a difference between the samples is proven to exist. Therefore, the goal of the tasting would be for a maximum of 17 participants to correctly detect a difference between the old and new recipe.

If so, the recipe modification has been successfully made and can be implemented. However, with at least 18 correct answers, the null hypothesis is rejected, which means that the adapted recipe needs to be revised as part of the product development or another alternative to methyl cellulose needs to be found.

6. Summary and results

The Chilean company "NotCo" is now distributing vegan substitute products not only in South America, but also in the United States of America. To make its products even more attractive to the markets, all artificial ingredients will be replaced by natural ingredients in its vegan burger "NotBurger". Therefore, a new recipe was developed to replace methyl cellulose with flaxseed. As all other plant-based ingredients remain unchanged, the taste, color and texture should not change in any noticeable way for the consumer.

To test this, a sensory panel composed of regular consumers of the "NotBurger" will be formed. After recruiting them through social networks, the tasting will take place in one day at the company's premises with 36 participants. The tasting booths have been set up and equipped according to the given guidelines. To determine whether there is a difference between the new and old recipe that can be recognized by the layman, a triangle test is performed.

In this test, each participant is presented with three samples, one of which is different from the other two. The task here is to recognize the different sample. All samples are marked with a random three-digit number to avoid the subconscious influence of classification. After all participants have filled out and handed in their questionnaire independently, the evaluation is performed. It has to be checked whether the null hypothesis "no difference" can be rejected or not. If it is rejected, the recipe without methylcellulose has to be revised. However, the objective is that the hypothesis is accepted and the flaxseed product can be launched on the market without further changes.

7. List of figures

8. Bibliography

Chen, F. L., Wei, Y. M., Zhang, B., & Ojokoh, A. O. (2010). System parameters and product properties response of soybean protein extruded at wide moisture range. *Journal of Food Engineering*, 208-212.

Fischer, J. (19. February 2020). *Utopia*. Von Methylcellulose (E461): Was du über das Verdickungsmittel wissen musst: https://utopia.de/ratgeber/methylcellulose-e-461-was-du-ueber-das-verdickungsmittel-wissen-musst/ abgerufen

Gardenia . (21. January 2023). Von Linum ustiatissimum : https://www.gardenia.net/plant/linum-lusitatissimum abgerufen

Hassan, J. (09. March 2021). *Business Wire*. Von NotCo Named to Fast Company's Annual List of the World's Most Innovative Companies: https://www.businesswire.com/news/home/20210309005794/en/NotCo-Named-to-Fast-Company%E2%80%99s-Annual-List-of-the-World%E2%80%99s-Most-Innovative-Companies abgerufen

Lebensmittelverband Deutschland. (28. Octubre 2022). Von Clean Labels: https://www.lebensmittelverband.de/de/lebensmittel/werbung/clean-labels abgerufen

Moggia, C. (2022). *Uso de herramientas estadísticas para la interpretación de datos.* Universidad de Talca: Notas de clase "Análisis sensorial para el desarrollo de productos".

Navarro, M. (2022). *Planificación de un ensayo sensorial.* Universidad de Talca: Notas de clase "Análisis sensorial para el desarrollo de productos".

NotCo. (28. October 2022). Von https://notco.com/cl/ abgerufen

Statistisches Bundesamt, D. (21. Julio 2020). *Vegetarische und vegane Lebensmittel: Produktion steigt im 1. Quartal 2020 um 37%.* Von https://www.destatis.de/DE/Presse/Pressemitteilungen/Zahl-der-Woche/2020/PD20_30_p002.html abgerufen

Uniflex. (28. October 2022). Von Flexible Verpackungen für Tiefkühlkost: https://www.uniflexpackaging.de/marktloesungen/tiefkuehlwaren_verpackung abgerufen

Vázquez-Rowe, I. (2020). A fine kettle of fish: the fishing industry and environmental impacts. *Current Opinion in Environmental Science & Health*, S. 1-5.

Vogt, C., & Teichmann, P. (23. Febrero 2021). *Migros*. Von Alles Wissenswerte über Tiefkühlkost: https://impuls.migros.ch/de/ernaehrung/ernaehrungswissen/umgang-mit-lebensmitteln/tiefkuehlkost abgerufen

Wang, H., Johnson, L. A., & Wang, T. (2004). Preparation of soy protein concentrate and isolate from extruded-expelled soybean meals. *J Amer Oil Chem Soc*, 713-717.

Wikipedia. (21. June 2022). Von NotCo: https://en.wikipedia.org/wiki/NotCo abgerufen

Wittek, P., Zeiler, N., Karbstein, H. P., & Emin, M. A. (2020). Analysis of the complex rheological properties of highly concentrated proteins with a closed cavity rheometer. *Applied Rheology*, 64-76.